AF457381

Contents

What Is Quesadilla?

A quesadilla is a Mexican cuisine dish, consisting of a thin dough or tortilla that is filled primarily with cheese, and sometimes meats, spices, and other fillings, and then cooked on a griddle or stove. Traditionally, a corn tortilla is used, but it can also be made with a flour tortilla.

A full quesadilla is made with two tortillas that hold a layer of cheese between them. A half is a single tortilla that has been filled with cheese and folded into a half-moon shape.

HISTORY OF THE QUESADILLA

Literally meaning "little cheesy thing," quesadillas originated in northern and central Mexico in the 16th century.

Corn tortillas were already popular among the Aztec people. They often stuffed them with squash and pumpkin and baked them in clay ovens as a sweet dessert. In 1521, Spanish settlers brought sheep, lambs, and cows with them to New Spain, thus introducing indigenous people to cheese and other dairy products. The indigenous people continued stuffing their tortillas with pumpkin and squash, but also added cheese to the mix. Thus, the quesadilla was born.

The quesadilla quickly increased in popularity, and to this day has remained a favorite dish in Mexican cuisine.

TIPS TO MAKE A QUESADILLA

PREPARE THE FILLING

Prepare the filling: Pick a few of the suggested filling ingredients above, enough to make 2 to 3 cups of total filling. If combining leftovers, warm them briefly in the microwave or in a skillet over medium heat. If using raw ingredients, cook before making quesadillas. Transfer the filling to a bowl and cover to keep warm.

MELT ½ TEASPOON OF BUTTER

OR OIL IN THE SKILLET

Ironically, the key to a crispy quesadilla is less fat in the pan, not more. Too much fat will make your quesadilla soggy instead of crispy. Use just enough to coat the bottom of your skillet—about

1/2 teaspoon of butter or oil. Warm it in the skillet over medium to medium-high heat.

ADD THE TORTILLA AND TOP WITH CHEESE

Lay one tortilla in the skillet and sprinkle all over with 1/2 cup of cheese. Don't feel obliged to use flour or corn. Expand your horizons to spinach or red pepper infused tortillas. If you have a little more time on your hands, make the tortillas yourself!

Tip: Double check that your tortilla is large enough to fit all of the filling into it. 9"–10" tortillas are usually best.

ADD THE FILLING

Spread roughly 1/2 cup of filling in a single layer over just half of the tortilla. Don't use too much or the filling will fall out as you try to eat it. Spreading the filling over half makes the quesadilla easier to fold, and adding it as the cheese melts gives the filling time to warm if it has cooled.

WATCH FOR THE CHEESE TO MELT

Once the cheese starts to melt, begin lifting a corner of the tortilla and checking the underside. When the cheese has completely melted and you see golden-brown spots on the underside of the tortilla, the quesadilla is ready.

Tip: Be patient! The quesadilla will grill better and a more even melt on medium heat.

FOLD THE QUESADILLA IN HALF

Use the spatula to fold the quesadilla in half, sandwiching the filling.

TRANSFER TO A CUTTING BOARD

AND SLICE INTO WEDGES

Slide the hot quesadilla onto a cutting board. If you are serving (or eating) the quesadilla immediately, slice into wedges. Using a pizza sliver always helps!

Tip: If you are not serving it immediately, slide the quesadilla onto a baking sheet and keep it in a 200 degree oven.

Tip: For optimal tastiness, only slice the quesadilla into wedges immediately before serving.

ENJOY, WIPE THE PAN CLEAN,

AND REPEAT!

Tip: When cooking for a crowd, be sure to continually adding butter to the pan or skillet for each quesadilla you make.

Tip: If you are making quesadillas for a large crowd, use a pancake skillet. You'll thank us—it will make things go a lot faster.

pare the filling: Pick a few of the suggested filling ingredients above, enough to make 2 to 3 cups of total filling. If combining leftovers, warm them briefly

One Day Quesadillas Meal Plan

Each of these recipes has 5 ingredients or less. To make these recipes dorm-friendly, skip the stove and iron your quesadilla.

Breakfast: Quesarito

This mashup uses a quesadilla as the shell of your breakfast burrito. The hearty eggs and avocado will keep you energized throughout the day.Y

Prep Time: 7 minutes

Cook Time: 5 minutes

Total Time: 12 minutes

Servings: 1

Ingredients:

2 medium tortilla shells

1/3 cup shredded cheese

1 avocado

3 tablespoons salsa

2 eggs

1 teaspoon butter

Directions:

1. Melt butter in a skillet on medium heat.

2. Place 1 tortilla shell on skillet and cover with shredded cheese.

3. Top with the other tortilla, and cook each side until golden brown.

4. While your quesadilla is cooking, scramble some eggs in a separate pan. Check out this recipe for normal scrambled eggs or this recipe for microwave scrambled eggs.

6. Scoop the avocado into a bowl with a spoon, and mash it with a fork

7. Top the quesadilla with the mashed avocado, eggs, and salsa.

8. Roll up and dig into your new breakfast favorite.

Lunch: Veggie Roll-up

Use a quesadilla instead of a plain tortilla to take your veggie wrap to the next level. This mashup will transform your boring, cold wrap into a warm, zesty meal.

Prep Time: 3 minutes

Cook Time: 6 minutes

Total Time: 9 minutes

Servings: 1

Ingredients:

2 medium tortilla shells

1/3 cup shredded cheese

2 tablespoons hummus (Choose a flavored hummus to add a lot of flavor with just a little effort.)

1 sliced portobello mushroom (or whichever veggies you like)

1 teaspoon butter

Directions:

1. Melt butter in a skillet on medium heat.

2. Place 1 tortilla shell on skillet and cover with shredded cheese.

3. Cover with the second tortilla and cook until each side is a golden brown.

4. Plate the quesadilla, and spread hummus and mushrooms (or other veggies) down the middle.

5. Roll up like a burrito. Bon appétit.

Dinner: Doritos Stuffed Chicken Quesadilla

Prep Time: 5 minutes

Cook Time: 15 minutes

Total Time: 20 minutes

Servings: 1

Ingredients:

2 medium flour tortillas

½ cup diced chicken breast

1/3 cup shredded cheese

1/3 can diced green chiles

5 crushed Doritos chips

2 tablespoons olive oil or butter

Directions:

1. Cook chicken in a pan with oil on medium high heat until it is white all the way though.

2. Melt butter in a pan on medium heat to coat it, and top with a tortilla.

3. Cover the tortilla with cheese, crushed Doritos, green chiles and chicken.

4. Top with the other tortilla, and cook until golden brown.

Enjoy!

Dessert: Raspberry Nutella Roll a la Mode

Don't think I would possibly forget about dessert. Just substitute the cheese with nutella.

Prep Time: 3 minutes

Cook Time: 3 minutes

Total Time: 6 minutes

Servings: 1

Ingredients:

2 medium tortilla shells

2 tablespoons nutella

2 tablespoons raspberry jam

1-2 scoops ice cream

1 teaspoon butter

Directions:

1. Melt butter in a skillet on medium heat.

2. Spread nutella on the side of one tortilla and raspberry jam on the other tortilla.

3. Place them on top of each other sandwich style, and heat on the pan.

4. Plate it, and top with ice cream.

QUESADILLA RECIPES

Whenever I hear the word "quesadilla" my mind automatically pictures a typical white-flour tortilla stuffed with chicken, cheese, and sometimes beans. And while that might sound kind of tasty, it's not all that healthy and definitely not very exciting. But after going on the hunt for some more creative variations of this dinnertime favorite, I found that you can fill quesadillas with just about anything as long as you have a tortilla on hand.

We bring you quesadillas stuffed with everything from quinoa, kale, black beans, spinach, feta cheese, tofu, avocado, peppers, tomatoes, and more. They're super easy to make and can be eaten for a full meal or sliced up and served as an appetizer to share amongst friends. Whichever way you slice it, it's guaranteed to be delicious and way healthier than your boring cheese quesadilla. Happy cooking, friends!

Chicken Quesadillas

Prepartion time

40 minutes

Ingredients

- 12 large flour tortillas
- 2 tablespoons olive oil
- 2 1/2 cups grated cheese (Monterey Jack is the best)
- 2 pounds skinless chicken breasts
- Salt and pepper
- 2 tablespoons taco or Cajun seasoning mix
- 1 large onion, cut in half and then into slices
- 1 green bell pepper, seeded and sliced into strips
- 1 red bell pepper, seeded and sliced into strips

- 1 yellow bell pepper
- 12 tablespoons butter, for frying

Pico de Gallo:

- 12 Roma tomatoes (slightly under ripe is fine)
- 3 yellow or red onions
- 2 cups fresh cilantro leaves
- 2 to 3 jalapenos
- 1 lime
- Salt

Instructions

1. Heat 1 tablespoon of the olive oil in a skillet over high heat.

2. Sprinkle the chicken with salt, pepper and taco seasoning.

3. Add the chicken to the skillet and saute over medium-high heat until done, about 4 minute per side.

4. Remove from the skillet and dice into cubes. Set aside.

5. Add the remaining 1 tablespoon olive oil to the skillet over high heat.

6. Throw in the onions and peppers and cook until the peppers have a few dark brown/black areas, 3 to 4 minutes.

7. Remove and set aside.

8. Sizzle 1/2 tablespoon of the butter in a separate skillet or griddle over medium heat and lay a flour tortilla in the skillet.

9. Then build the quesadillas by laying grated cheese on the bottom tortilla, and then arranging the chicken and cooked peppers.

10. Top with a little more grated cheese and top with a second tortilla.

11. When the tortilla is golden on the first side, carefully flip the quesadilla to the other side, adding another 1/2 tablespoon butter to the skillet at the same time.

12. Continue cooking until the second side is golden.

13. Repeat with the remaining tortillas and fillings.

14. Cut each quesadilla into wedges and serve with Pico de Gallo.

Pico de Gallo:

1. Dice up equal quantities of tomatoes and onions.

2. Roughly chop the cilantro.

3. Now, slice 1 or 2 jalapenos in half.

4. With a spoon, scrape out the seeds. (If you like things spicy, leave in some of the white membranes.)

5. Dice the jalapenos very finely; you want a hint of heat and jalapeno flavor, but you don't want to cause any fires.

6. Now dump the four ingredients into a bowl.

7. Slice the lime in half and squeeze the juice from half the lime into the bowl.

8. Sprinkle with salt, and stir together until combined.

9. Be sure to taste the pico de gallo and adjust the seasonings, adding salt or more diced jalapeno if needed.

Chicken, Chili, and Cheese Quesadillas

Prepartion time

50 minutes

Ingredients

Quesadillas:

- 12 corn tortillas, preferably white
- 6 ounces Cheddar, Monterey Jack or Colby cheese, thinly sliced
- 1 tablespoon chopped pickled jalapenos
- 1 cup shredded cooked chicken (about 3 ounces)
- 4 tablespoons (1/2 stick) unsalted butter

Topping and Salsa:

- 1 pound vine-ripened tomatoes (about 2 tomatoes)
- 1/4 small red onion
- 2 to 3 tablespoons chopped cilantro
- Hot sauce such as chipotle or Mexican green chili sauce to taste (1/2 teaspoon)
- Kosher salt
- 1 Hass avocado, halved, seeded and sliced

Instructions

1. Lay 6 tortillas on the work surface, and divide the cheese, jalapenos and chicken among the tortillas. (It's best to leave about an inch border on the edge of the tortilla uncovered to allow for the spread of the melting cheese.)

2. Top with remaining tortillas and press gently to seal.

3. Melt 1 tablespoon butter in a small skillet.

4. Carefully place a quesadilla in the skillet and fry, turning once, until golden and little bubbles appear on both sides, 4 to 5 minutes in all.

5. Repeat with the remaining quesadillas, wiping out the pan between batches if the butter burns.

6. While the quesadillas cook, make the salsa: Halve the tomatoes and grate them on the largest holes of a box grater into a bowl, discarding the skins.

7. Grate the onion into the tomato and stir in the cilantro, hot sauce and salt, to taste.

8. Cut quesadillas into 4 wedges with a pizza wheel or knife and serve with the salsa and avocado.

Waffled Chorizo-Cheese Quesadilla

Prepartion time

45 minutes

Ingredients

- 1 lime, juiced
- 1/4 small red onion, thinly sliced
- Pinch kosher salt
- 1 teaspoon vegetable oil, plus more brushing tortillas

- 2 ounces fresh chorizo, removed from casings
- Four 6- to 8-inch flour tortillas
- 2/3 cup shredded Cheddar
- Salsa, sour cream and chopped avocado, for serving

Instructions

1. Combine the lime juice, onions and salt in a small nonreactive bowl, tossing occasionally.

2. Let sit at room temperature until the onions are pink, about 15 minutes.

3. Heat the oil in a medium nonstick skillet over medium-high heat.

4. Add the chorizo and cook, breaking up with a wooden spoon, until browned, about 3 minutes.

5. Preheat a waffle iron to medium-high.

6. Brush one side of 2 tortillas with oil and lay dry-side up on a work surface.

7. Scatter each with 1/3 cup cheese, then the pickled onions. Sandwich with the remaining tortillas and brush the tops with oil.

8. Place 1 quesadilla in the waffle iron, close gently (don't push down) and cook until golden brown and the cheese is melted, 4 to 6 minutes.

9. Repeat with the remaining quesadilla.

10. Cut the quesadillas into wedges and top with the chorizo. Serve with salsa, sour cream and avocado.

Southwest Quesadilla with Cilantro-Lime Sour Cream

Prepartion time

30 minutes

Ingredients

- 2 tablespoons olive oil, plus extra for griddle
- 1 small red bell pepper, diced
- 1/2 red onion, diced
- 3/4 cup corn kernels, (about 1 ear)
- 2 teaspoons red pepper flakes
- 1 teaspoon ground cumin

- Salt and freshly ground black pepper
- 1/2 cup freshly chopped cilantro leaves
- Four 10-inch "burrito size" flour tortillas
- One 16-ounce can refried black beans
- 1 cup grated Pepper Jack cheese

Lime-Cilantro Sour Cream:

- 1/2 cup sour cream
- 1/4 cup freshly chopped cilantro leaves
- 1/2 lime, juiced
- Pinch salt

Instructions

1. In a large skillet, heat oil over medium-high heat.

2. Saute red pepper and onion until soft, about 5 minutes.

3. Add corn, red pepper flakes, cumin, and salt and pepper to taste.

4. Toss to incorporate and saute for 3 minutes.

5. Transfer to a bowl and add the cilantro.

6. Preheat a long, 2-burner cast iron griddle, or a large saute pan over medium heat.

7. Lay 2 tortillas on a work surface and spread each evenly with refried black beans.

8. Place tortillas, bean side up, on the griddle (begin with 1 if using a saute pan).

9. Sprinkle onion-red pepper mixture evenly over the top of each, then sprinkle evenly with the cheese.

10. Cover with another tortilla coated with refried black beans and cook until cheese melts, about 4 minutes.

11. Flip quesadillas to toast the other side.

12. Slice each quesadilla into 8 wedges, sprinkle with cilantro, and serve with Lime-Cilantro Sour Cream.

Purslane Quesadillas

Prepartion time

20 minutes

Ingredients

- 4 ounces purslane
- Four 8-inch flour tortillas
- 8 ounces low-moisture whole milk mozzarella or Oaxacan cheese, coarsely grated
- 8 teaspoons prepared salsa verde
- 4 teaspoons unsalted butter

Instructions

1. Tear the purslane into 2- or 3-inch pieces, stripping the little shoots from the main stems; discard the woodiest pieces.

2. Lay the tortillas on your work surface.

3. Sprinkle some cheese on half of each tortilla, leaving 1/2-inch border.

4. Put some purslane on top of the cheese, and drizzle about 2 teaspoons of the salsa verde on top.

5. Top the purslane with the remaining cheese. Fold the tortillas in half.

6. Heat a medium nonstick skillet over medium heat.

7. Add 2 teaspoons of the butter and melt until the foam just about subsides.

8. Put in 2 of the tortillas and cook, pressing lightly with a spatula once or twice, until the underside is golden brown, about 2 minutes.

9. Flip, and cook until the second side is brown and the cheese is melted, about 2 more minutes.

10. Transfer the tortillas to a cutting board.

11. Wipe out the skillet.

12. Repeat with the remaining butter and tortillas, lowering the heat a bit if the butter or tortilla browns too quickly.

13. Use a pizza wheel or sharp knife to cut the quesadillas into wedges and serve immediately.

Dessert Quesadilla

Prepartion time

30 minutes

Ingredients

- Four 8-inch flour tortillas, cut in half
- 1 large egg, beaten
- 1/2 cup chocolate hazelnut spread
- Eight 1/4-inch-thick slices of fresh fruit such as banana, strawberry or plum or 8 marshmallows
- 3 tablespoons unsalted butter, melted
- Confectioners' sugar, for dusting

Instructions

1. Lay 1 tortilla half on a clean work surface with the rounded side closest to you.

2. Brush the edges of the tortilla with egg.

3. Place 1 tablespoon of chocolate hazelnut spread in the center of the tortilla and place a piece of fruit or marshmallow on top.

4. Fold one side of the tortilla half way over the filling so that the corner is in the 6-o'clock position, press to seal.

5. Fold the other side over the filling so that the two edges overlap slightly and the corner is also in the 6-o'clock position, press to seal.

6. The quesadilla will look like a triangle-shaped hand pie.

7. Repeat with the remaining tortilla halves and fillings.

8. Melt half the butter in a large nonstick skillet over medium heat and cook half of the

quesadillas until deep golden brown, about 2 minutes per side.

9. Transfer to a paper towel-lined plate.

10. Wipe the skillet clean and repeat with remaining butter and quesadillas.

11. Dust with confectioners' sugar before serving.

Chorizo and Shrimp Quesadillas with Smoky Guacamole

Prepartion time

25 minutes

Ingredients

- 2 ripe Haas avocados
- 1 lime, juiced
- A couple pinches salt
- 1/4 cup sour cream, 3 rounded tablespoonfuls
- 2 chipotle peppers in adobo, available in cans on specialty food aisle in Mexican section
- 1/2 pound chorizo sausage, sliced thin on an angle

- 1 tablespoon extra virgin olive oil, plus some for drizzling
- 1 clove garlic, cracked away from skin and crushed
- 12 large shrimp, peeled and deveined, tails removed, ask for easy-peels at fish counter
- Salt and freshly ground black pepper
- 4 (12- inch) flour tortillas
- 1/2 pound, 2 cups, shredded pepper Jack cheese

Instructions

1. Cut avocados all the way around with a sharp knife.

2. Scoop out the pit, then spoon avocado flesh away from skin into a food processor.

3. Add the juice of 1 lime, a couple of pinches salt, sour cream and chipotles in adobo.

4. Pulse guacamole until smooth.

5. Transfer to a serving bowl.

6. Heat a 12-inch nonstick skillet over medium high heat.

7. Brown chorizo 2 to 3 minutes, then remove from pan.

8. Add oil, garlic, then shrimp.

9. Season shrimp with salt and pepper and cook shrimp until pink, 2 or 3 minutes.

10. Transfer shrimp to a cutting board and coarsely chop.

11. Add a drizzle of oil to the pan and a large tortilla.

12. Cook tortilla 30 seconds, then turn. Cover 1/2 of the tortilla with a couple of handfuls of cheese.

13. Arrange a layer of chorizo and shrimp over the cheese and fold tortilla over.

14. Press down gently with a spatula and cook tortilla a minute or so on each side to melt cheese and crisp.

15. Remove quesadilla to large cutting board and repeat with remaining ingredients.

16. Cut each quesadilla into 5 wedges and transfer to plates with your spatula.

17. Top wedges of quesadillas with liberal amounts of smoky guacamole.

The Greatest Quesadilla

Prepartion time

30 minutes

Ingredients

- 1 cup grated white Cheddar cheese
- 1 cup grated Monterey Jack cheese
- 1 cup grated pepper jack cheese
- 6 tablespoons salted butter
- Six 8-inch flour tortillas

- Pinch of kosher salt
- Pinch of freshly ground black pepper
- 2 Roma tomatoes, diced
- One 4-ounce can diced green chiles, drained
- 9 fresh cilantro sprigs, for garnish

Instructions

1. Toss together the Cheddar, Monterey Jack and pepper jack in a bowl; set aside.

2. Heat 2 tablespoons of the butter in large skillet over medium heat.

3. Place a single tortilla in the skillet.

4. Sprinkle a little less than a third of the cheese blend over the tortilla.

5. Sprinkle with salt and pepper.

6. Add about a third of the diced tomato and a third of the chiles.

7. Sprinkle a touch more cheese over the whole thing and gently top and press with a second tortilla.

8. Cook until golden on the bottom, about 3 minutes.

9. Carefully flip the quesadilla to the other side.

10. Continue cooking until the second side is golden, 3 to 4 minutes more.

11. Repeat with the remaining ingredients.

12. Slice each quesadilla into wedges and garnish with cilantro sprigs.

Stewed Chicken, Refried Beans and Oaxaca Cheese Quesadillas

Prepartion time

30 minutes

Ingredients

- One 15-ounce can fire-roasted tomatoes
- 2 teaspoons chili powder
- 1 clove garlic, finely grated
- Kosher salt and freshly ground black pepper
- One 8-ounce boneless skinless chicken breast
- Four 10-inch (burrito size) flour tortillas

- 2 cups shredded Oaxaca cheese
- 1 cup refried beans
- 2 tablespoons unsalted butter
- Guacamole, salsa, chopped scallions and sour cream, for serving

Instructions

1. Combine the tomatoes, chili powder, garlic, 2/3 cup water and 1/2 teaspoon salt in a small saucepan.

2. Bring to a simmer over medium heat and cook, breaking up the tomatoes with a spoon, for 10 minutes.

3. Add the chicken breast, nestling it in the sauce, and simmer, flipping once, until cooked through, 8 to 9 minutes per side.

4. Transfer the chicken to a plate, shred it, and return it to the sauce.

5. Season with salt and pepper.

6. Lay a tortilla on a work surface and top evenly with 1/2 cup Oaxaca cheese.

7. Add a quarter of the shredded chicken and tomato sauce and a quarter of the beans.

8. Fold the tortilla in half to enclose the fillings. Repeat with the remaining tortillas and ingredients.

9. Melt 1/2 tablespoon butter in a large nonstick or cast-iron skillet over medium heat.

10. Cook one of the quesadillas, flipping once, until golden brown and the cheese is melted, about 3 minutes per side.

11. Remove to a cutting board and repeat with the remaining quesadillas.

12. Cut into triangles and serve with the guacamole, salsa, scallions and sour cream.

Chicken and Roasted Poblano Quesadilla with Avocado Cream

Prepartion time

1 hour 15 minutes

Ingredients

- 2 boneless, skinless chicken thighs
- 3/4 teaspoon ground cumin
- Kosher salt
- 1/2 cup sour cream
- Finely grated zest and juice of 1 lime, plus lime wedges, for serving
- 1/2 firm, ripe avocado, pitted and peeled
- 1 small poblano chile, halved lengthwise, stemmed and seeded
- 4 scallions, thinly sliced

- 2 cups shredded Mexican cheese blend (8 ounces)
- 1 small clove garlic, finely grated
- 8 small corn tortillas
- 4 tablespoons vegetable oil
- Salsa, for serving

Instructions

1. Prick the chicken all over with a fork and put in a medium bowl.

2. Rub the cumin and 3/4 teaspoon salt into the chicken.

3. Add 1/4 cup of the sour cream and half the lime zest and juice and mix until the chicken is coated.

4. Let sit at room temperature for 15 minutes.

5. Blend the avocado, remaining 1/4 cup sour cream, remaining lime zest and juice, 3 tablespoons water and 1/2 teaspoon salt in a blender until very smooth; refrigerate until ready to use.

6. Meanwhile, preheat the broiler.

7. Line a rimmed baking sheet with foil.

8. Put the poblanos skin-side up on the prepared baking sheet and broil until the skin is wrinkled and charred in spots, 2 to 3 minutes.

9. Transfer the poblanos to a medium bowl, cover with plastic wrap and let steam for 5 minutes.

10. Run the poblanos under cold water and remove and discard the skin.

11. Cut the poblanos into small bite-size pieces and return them to the bowl.

12. Transfer the chicken to the baking sheet and broil, turning once, until browned in spots and cooked through, 4 to 5 minutes per side.

13. Let cool for a few minutes.

14. Cut it into small bite-size pieces.

15. Add the chicken and half of the scallions to the bowl with the poblanos and toss to combine.

16. Combine the cheese and garlic in a small bowl.

17. Top 4 tortillas with 1/4 cup of the cheese mixture, one-quarter of the chicken-poblano mixture then 1/4 cup more cheese mixture.

18. Top each with 1 of the remaining 4 tortillas and press lightly.

19. Heat 1 tablespoon of the oil in a large nonstick skillet over medium heat.

20. Add 1 quesadilla to the skillet and cook, turning once, until it is golden and the cheese is melted, 2 to 3 minutes per side.

21. Transfer to a baking sheet or large plate and repeat with the remaining oil and quesadillas.

22. Cut each quesadilla into quarters and sprinkle with the remaining scallions.

23. Serve with a dollop of the avocado cream, lime wedges and salsa on the side.

Meatloaf Quesadillas

Prepartion time

40 minutes

Ingredients

- 1 small head broccoli, cut into small florets, stems reserved
- 1 carrot, thinly sliced
- 2 limes (1 juiced, 1 cut into wedges)

- 1/2 cup fresh cilantro, roughly chopped
- 1/4 cup chopped pickled jalapeno peppers, plus 3 tablespoons of the brine
- 1/4 cup extra-virgin olive oil, plus more if needed
- 3 plum tomatoes, diced
- 1/4 small white onion, diced
- 3 cups crumbled cold leftover Slow-Cooker Meatloaf
- 3 burrito-size flour tortillas
- 2 cups shredded Mexican cheese blend or sharp cheddar (about 8 ounces)
- Sour cream, for serving

Slow-Cooker Meatloaf

- 2 1/4 pounds ground meatloaf mix (a combination of beef, pork and veal)
- 1 cup panko breadcrumbs
- 2 large eggs
- 1 1/4 cups ketchup
- 2 tablespoons Worcestershire sauce
- 4 scallions, finely chopped
- 2 tablespoons chopped fresh parsley, plus more for topping
- 2 teaspoons chopped fresh thyme
- Kosher salt and freshly ground pepper
- 12 ounces small fingerling potatoes, halved lengthwise

- 3 carrots, sliced 1 inch thick
- 1/4 cup low-sodium chicken broth
- 2 tablespoons packed light brown sugar

Instructions

1. Preheat the oven to 400 degrees F.
2. Put the broccoli florets in a microwave-safe bowl and add 2 tablespoons water.
3. Cover with plastic wrap and microwave until tender, about 3 minutes; set aside.
4. Meanwhile, trim the broccoli stems and peel into wide ribbons using a vegetable peeler; transfer to a large bowl.

5. Add the carrot, half each of the lime juice, cilantro and jalapenos, the brine and 3 tablespoons olive oil; toss.

6. Drain the florets and rinse under cold water; add to the salad and toss.

7. Combine the tomatoes, onion and remaining lime juice, cilantro and jalapenos in a bowl. Mix half of the salsa with the meatloaf.

8. Divide the meatloaf mixture among the tortillas, spreading it on one side.

9. Top with the cheese, then fold the tortillas in half over the filling.

10. Heat the remaining 1 tablespoon olive oil in a large nonstick skillet over medium-high heat.

11. Working in batches and re-oiling the skillet as needed, cook the quesadillas until golden, 1 to 2 minutes per side.

12. Transfer to a baking sheet and bake until the cheese melts, 5 minutes.

13. Cut the quesadillas into wedges and serve with the sour cream, remaining salsa, lime wedges and broccoli salad.

Slow-Cooker Meatloaf

1. Combine the meatloaf mix, panko, eggs, 3/4 cup ketchup, 1 tablespoon Worcestershire sauce, the scallions, parsley, thyme, 1 teaspoon salt and a few grinds of pepper in a large bowl; mix with your hands until just combined. Form into a 5-by-9-inch loaf.

2. Transfer the meatloaf to a 6-quart slow cooker.

3. Scatter the potatoes and carrots over and around the meatloaf.

4. Pour in the chicken broth.

5. Cover the slow cooker and cook 8 hours on low or 4 hours on high.

6. When the meatloaf is done, skim off any excess fat from the juices in the slow cooker.

7. Combine the remaining 1/2 cup ketchup, 1 tablespoon Worcestershire sauce and the brown sugar in a small bowl, then whisk in 1/4 cup juices from the slow cooker.

8. Brush the top of the meatloaf with the ketchup mixture.

9. Cover the slow cooker and let the meatloaf rest, 10 minutes.

10. Remove the meatloaf from the slow cooker and slice in half.

11. Serve half with the vegetables; top with more parsley.

Ham, Apple and Cheese Quesadilla

Prepartion time

30 minutes

Ingredients

- Eight 6-inch whole wheat tortillas
- Cooking spray or olive oil, for oiling tortillas

- 1 tablespoon spicy brown or Dijon mustard
- 1 cup shredded low-sodium Swiss (4 ounces)
- 4 ounces very thinly sliced low-sodium lean Black Forest or Virginia ham
- 1/2 small red onion, extra thinly sliced
- Freshly ground black pepper
- 1 1/2 tablespoons no-sugar-added apple butter, plus more for topping, optional
- 2 small apples, cut into thin sticks (red and green)
- Lemon juice and ground cinnamon for tossing

Instructions

1. Preheat the oven to 200 degrees F.

2. Spray 4 of the tortillas with cooking spray (or brush with olive oil).

3. Lay the oiled tortillas on a large cutting board oiled-side down.

4. Brush with the mustard and sprinkle with about half of the cheese.

5. Top each evenly with a thin layer of ham, onions and some pepper, and then finish with the remaining cheese.

6. Brush the apple butter evenly on the remaining tortillas.

7. Place one apple-butter tortilla on top of a ham-and-cheese tortilla (filling sides in), and firmly press the tortillas together to make a quesadilla.

8. Heat a large nonstick skillet over medium heat.

9. Lay a quesadilla oiled-side down in the pan and cook until golden brown and the cheese starts to melt, about 2 minutes.

10. Spray the top of the quesadilla with cooking spray, turn and cook until the other side browns and the cheese is melted, 2 to 3 minutes more.

11. Transfer to a baking sheet and keep warm in the oven.

12. Repeat with the remaining quesadillas.

13. Cut the quesadillas into 4 wedges and arrange on plates.

14. Toss the apples with lemon and juice and cinnamon to taste.

15. Serve with the apple slices.

Shrimp Quesadilla

Prepartion time

1 hour 20 minutes

Ingredients

- 8 ounces pepper jack cheese
- Six 16-20 count unpeeled shrimp, deveined
- Olive oil, for drizzling
- Kosher salt and freshly ground black pepper
- 2 tablespoons mayonnaise

- 2 large flour tortillas
- 1/4 cup chopped roasted red pepper
- 1/4 cup chopped fresh cilantro leaves

Instructions

1. Place cheese in freezer for around 45 minutes.

2. Meanwhile, preheat oven to 400 degrees F.

3. Drizzle shrimp with olive oil in a large bowl.

4. Sprinkle with salt and pepper and toss to coat.

5. Spread on a baking sheet and bake, rotating once, until just cooked through, 7 to 9 minutes.

6. When shrimp are cool enough to handle, remove and discard peels and tails. Cut shrimp into thirds.

7. Shred cheese using the large holes on a box grater.

8. Spread 1 tablespoon mayonnaise on one side of a tortilla. Place tortilla, mayo-side down, in a large skillet.

9. Sprinkle half the cheese evenly over the top of the entire tortilla, then turn heat on to medium-low heat.

10. While pan is heating, sprinkle half of the chopped shrimp, half of the roasted red peppers and half of the cilantro on one half of the tortilla, leaving the other half with just cheese.

11. Let quesadilla cook, checking that the bottom of the tortilla doesn't burn, until cheese is mostly melted, 3 to 5 minutes.

12. Remove skillet from heat and carefully fold the quesadilla in half like a book, folding the cheese side over the toppings.

13. Place quesadilla on a plate and let rest 5 minutes. Repeat with second tortilla and ingredients.

14. Cut into wedges before serving.

Grilled Steak, Chipotle and Pepper Jack Quesadillas

Prepartion time

45 minutes

Ingredients

- 1 clove garlic, minced
- 1/4 teaspoon ground cumin
- Juice of half lime
- Juice of half orange
- Kosher salt
- 8 ounces cleaned and trimmed skirt steak
- Olive oil, for oiling the grill grates
- Four 10-inch (burrito size) flour tortillas
- 2 cups shredded pepper-jack cheese

- 1 to 2 chipotle in adobo, chopped, plus 1 to 2 tablespoons sauce
- 2 tablespoons unsalted butter
- Guacamole, salsa, chopped scallions and sour cream, for serving

Instructions

1. Preheat an outdoor grill over medium.
2. Whisk the garlic, cumin, lime and oranges juices and 1/2 teaspoon salt together in a medium bowl.
3. Add the steak, coat well in the mixture and let marinade for 10 minutes.
4. Lightly oil the grill grates.

5. Grill the steak, flipping once, until medium rare, 2 to 6 minutes per side depending on the thickness.

6. Remove to a cutting board and let rest 5 minutes.

7. Slice the steak against the grain and reserve.

8. Lay a tortilla on a work surface and top evenly with 1/2 cup pepper-jack cheese.

9. Add 1/4 of the steak and some chopped chipotle in adobo and sauce.

10. Fold the tortilla in half to enclose fillings.

11. Repeat with remaining tortillas and ingredients.

12. Melt 1/2 tablespoon butter in a large nonstick or cast-iron skillet over medium heat.

13. Cook the quesadilla, flipping once, until the cheese is melted and it is golden brown on both sides, about 3 minutes per side.

14. Remove to a cutting board and repeat with the remaining quesadillas.

15. Cut into triangles and serve with guacamole, salsa, scallions and sour cream.

Easy Chicken-Mushroom Quesadillas

Prepartion time

28 minutes

Ingredients

- 1 tablespoon canola oil
- 1 large onion, chopped (about 2 cups)
- 8 ounces white button mushrooms, (about 3 cups)
- 3 cloves garlic, minced
- 2 cups cooked chopped skinless, boneless chicken breast (1 breast half)
- 1 teaspoon ground cumin
- 1 teaspoon chili powder
- 1 teaspoon dried oregano
- 2 cups baby spinach leaves, sliced into ribbons

- 1/2 teaspoon salt
- 1/4 teaspoon fresh ground black pepper
- 4 (10-inch) whole-grain flour tortillas
- 1 cup shredded Mexican cheese mix or Cheddar
- 1/2 cup salsa
- 1/4 cup reduced-fat sour cream

Instructions

1. Heat the oil in a large skillet over a medium heat.

2. Add the onions and mushrooms and cook until the mushroom water is evaporated and they begin to brown, 5 to 7 minutes.

3. Add the garlic and cook for 1 minute more.

4. Add chicken, cumin, chili powder and oregano and stir until all spices are incorporated.

5. Add spinach, salt and pepper and cook until spinach is wilted, about 2 minutes.

6. Lay 1 tortilla on a flat work surface and sprinkle with 1/4 cup shredded cheese.

7. Spoon 1/2 chicken and vegetable mixture on top of cheese, then top with an additional 1/4 cup cheese.

8. Top with another flour tortilla. Heat a large nonstick skillet with cooking spray over medium heat.

9. Carefully place 1 quesadilla in pan and cook 3 minutes.

10. Using a large spatula, gently flip quesadilla and cook an additional 3 minutes until lightly browned and cheese is melted.

11. Repeat with second quesadilla.

12. Slice each quesadilla into quarters. Place 2 quarters on a plate with 1 tablespoon sour cream and 2 tablespoons salsa.

Chicken and Pepper Jack Quesadillas with Cilantro Slaw

Prepartion time

30 minutes

Ingredients

- 1 8-ounce package shredded coleslaw mix (about 4 cups)
- Kosher salt
- Juice of 1 lime
- 1 small clove garlic, finely chopped
- 1/2 cup packed fresh cilantro (leaves and tender stems), chopped
- 2 tablespoons vegetable oil
- Freshly ground pepper
- 4 burrito-size tortillas

- 8 ounces pepper jack cheese, shredded (about 2 cups)
- 1 cup chopped rotisserie chicken, skin removed
- 2 tablespoons unsalted butter
- 1/2 small head iceberg lettuce, shredded (about 4 cups)
- Mexican crema or sour cream, for topping

Instructions

1. Toss the coleslaw mix with 1/2 teaspoon salt in a large bowl and set aside.

2. Whisk the lime juice, garlic, cilantro, vegetable oil, 1/4 teaspoon salt and a few grinds of pepper in a small bowl.

3. Lay out the tortillas and sprinkle the cheese on half of each.

4. Season the chicken with salt and pepper and layer on top of the cheese.

5. Fold the tortillas in half. Heat 1 tablespoon butter in a large nonstick skillet over medium heat.

6. Add 2 quesadillas and cook, turning once, until browned and crisp and the cheese is melted, 5 to 7 minutes.

7. Transfer to a cutting board and repeat with the remaining butter and quesadillas.

8. Cut the quesadillas into wedges and divide among plates.

9. Add the lettuce and lime dressing to the coleslaw mix, toss to combine and season with salt and pepper.

10. Add to the plates and drizzle the quesadillas with the crema.

Bacon, Date and Manchego Quesadillas

Prepartion time

40 minutes

Ingredients

For the quesadillas:

- 12 slices bacon

- 4 10-inch flour tortillas
- 2 cups shredded manchego cheese (about 8 ounces)
- 5 dates, pitted and julienned
- 2 tablespoons extra-virgin olive oil

For the pistachio cream:

- 1/2 cup salted pistachios
- 1 teaspoon red pepper flakes
- 1 clove garlic, roughly chopped
- Juice of 1/2 lemon
- 2 cups spinach
- 1/4 cup extra-virgin olive oil

- Kosher salt and freshly ground pepper
- 1 cup Mexican crema or sour cream

Instructions

1. Preheat the oven to 400 degrees F.

2. Arrange the bacon slices side by side on a parchment-lined baking sheet and bake until browned and crisp, 15 to 18 minutes.

3. Drain on paper towels.

4. Meanwhile, make the pistachio cream: Combine the pistachios, red pepper flakes, garlic, lemon juice and spinach in a food processor and pulse until chopped; with the motor running, slowly stream in the olive oil until incorporated.

5. Season with salt and pepper and process 5 more seconds.

6. Pour the mixture into a bowl and whisk in the crema; set aside.

7. Assemble the quesadillas: On 1 half of each tortilla, layer 1/2 cup cheese, 3 slices bacon and a few date slices.

8. Fold the tortillas in half to cover the filling.

9. Heat 1 tablespoon olive oil in a nonstick skillet over medium heat.

10. Add 2 quesadillas and cook until golden on both sides and gooey in the middle, 4 to 5 minutes per side.

11. Repeat with the remaining 2 quesadillas, adding the remaining 1 tablespoon oil to the pan.

12. Cut each quesadilla into 4 triangles; serve with the pistachio cream.

Bacon and Hash Brown "Quesadilla" with Eggs

Prepartion time

1 hour 15 minutes

Ingredients

- 2 large russet potatoes (2 pounds), scrubbed
- Kosher salt and freshly ground black pepper

- 4 tablespoons canola oil, plus more for brushing
- 2 large Spanish onions, halved and thinly sliced
- 1 poblano chile, roasted and finely diced
- 1 tablespoon plus 2 teaspoons ancho chile powder
- 13 pound thick-cut bacon, diced
- 12 (6-inch) flour tortillas
- 2 12 cups grated Monterey Jack cheese
- 2 tablespoons unsalted butter
- 4 large eggs
- Fresh Tomato Salsa, recipe follows
- 2 tablespoons finely chopped fresh chives

Fresh Tomato Salsa:

• 2 ripe beefsteak tomatoes or 4 ripe plum tomatoes, diced

• 12 red onion, halved and thinly sliced

• 1 jalapeno, finely diced

• 2 tablespoons fresh lime juice

• 2 tablespoons canola oil

• 2 teaspoons honey

• 2 tablespoons finely chopped fresh cilantro

• Kosher salt and freshly ground black pepper

Instructions

1. Preheat the oven to 425 degrees F.

2. Heat 2 tablespoons of the oil in a large saute pan over medium heat.

3. Add the onions, season with salt and pepper, and cook, stirring occasionally, until golden brown and caramelized, about 30 minutes.

4. Heat the remaining 2 tablespoons oil in a large nonstick saute pan over high heat, add the potatoes, and cook until golden brown.

5. Stir in the onions, poblano, and 1 tablespoon of the ancho powder, season with salt and pepper, and cook until just warmed through, about 2 minutes.

6. Cook the bacon in a skillet over medium heat until browned and crisp, about 8 minutes.

7. Scoop out and transfer to a plate lined with paper towels to drain.

8. Lay out 8 of the tortillas on a work surface.

9. Divide the hash browns, bacon, and cheese among the tortillas.

10. Stack half of the tortillas on top of the remaining topped ones to create 4 double stacks.

11. Top each with one of the remaining 4 tortillas.

12. Brush the tops with a little oil and sprinkle with the remaining 2 teaspoons ancho powder.

13. Transfer the quesadillas to a large baking sheet and bake until golden brown and the cheese has melted, 8 to 10 minutes.

14. When the quesadillas are nearly ready, melt the butter in a large nonstick saute pan over medium heat.

15. Carefully crack the eggs into the pan, season with salt and pepper, and cook until the whites are set but the yolks are still runny, about 2 minutes.

16. Top each quesadilla with a fried egg, some of the tomato salsa, and a sprinkling of chives.

Fresh Tomato Salsa:

1. Combine all of the ingredients in a bowl and let sit at room temperature for at least 15 minutes before serving.

Asparagus, Bell Pepper and Mozzarella Quesadillas

Prepartion time

35 minutes

Ingredients

- 1 bunch medium asparagus woody stems trimmed and bottom 1/3 of the stalk peeled (about 1 pound),
- 2 tablespoons olive oil
- Kosher salt and freshly ground black pepper
- 2 red bell peppers, cut into 1/4-inch thick strips
- Four 10-inch (burrito size) flour tortillas

- 2 cups shredded Mozzarella
- 2 tablespoons unsalted butter

For Serving:

- Guacamole
- salsa
- chopped scallions
- sour cream for serving

Instructions

1. Arrange the asparagus in a microwave-safe dish, cover and microwave on high until crisp-tender, about 2 minutes. (If you don?t have a

microwave, you can steam the asparagus instead.)

2. Brush asparagus with 1 tablespoon of the oil.

3. Heat a grill pan over medium heat.

4. Grill the asparagus, flipping occasionally, until tender and lightly charred, about 5 minutes.

5. Cut asparagus in half crosswise and then slice on the bias into 1-inch pieces.

6. Sprinkle with salt and pepper.

7. Heat the remaining 1 tablespoon of oil in a large skillet over medium-high heat.

8. Add the peppers and cook, stirring frequently, until tender and slightly charred, 8 to 10 minutes.

9. Transfer to a bowl and stir in 1/2 teaspoon salt and a few grinds of pepper.

10. Lay a tortilla on a work surface and top evenly with 1/2 cup shredded cheese.

11. Add 1/4 of the asparagus and 1/4 of the peppers.

12. Fold tortilla in half to enclose fillings. Repeat with remaining tortillas and ingredients.

13. Melt 1/2 tablespoon of the butter in a large non-stick or cast-iron skillet over medium heat.

14. Cook the quesadilla, flipping once, until the cheese is melted and it is golden brown on both sides, about 3 minutes per side.

15. Remove to a cutting board and repeat with the remaining quesadillas.

16. Cut into triangles and serve topped with guacamole, salsa, chopped scallions and sour cream.

Cheesy Italian Beef Quesadillas

Prepartion time

20 minutes

Ingredients

- 4 large flour tortillas
- 1/2 pound provolone cheese, thinly sliced
- 1 pound good-quality roast beef, shaved very thin

- 1 cup jarred fire-roasted bell peppers, drained and julienned
- 2 tablespoons extra-virgin olive oil
- Garlic salt
- Mild giardiniera relish, for serving

Instructions

1. Heat a large nonstick skillet over medium heat.
2. On one half of a tortilla, layer some provolone, then a layer of beef, then some roasted peppers.
3. Fold in half to cover the lling.
4. Repeat to make 3 more quesadillas.

5. Add 1 tablespoon olive oil to the skillet.

6. Add 2 quesadillas and cook until golden on the outside and gooey in the middle, 4 to 6 minutes per side.

7. Slide out of the pan and sprinkle lightly with garlic salt.

8. Repeat with the remaining 2 quesadillas.

9. Cut into wedges and serve with giardiniera relish.

Fire-Grilled Chicken Quesadilla

Prepartion time

40 minutes

Ingredients

Quesadilla:

- 3 ounces boneless, skinless chicken breast
- Kosher salt and freshly ground black pepper
- 1/3 onion, sliced
- 1/3 green bell pepper, sliced
- 1 tablespoon grapeseed oil
- Two 6-inch flour tortillas
- 2 ounces shredded Monterey Jack
- 2 ounces shredded Cheddar

Salsa:

- 1/3 onion, diced
- 1/3 tomato, diced
- 1/2 lime, juiced
- 1/3 bunch fresh cilantro, chopped
- Kosher salt and freshly ground black pepper
- 2 teaspoons butter
- 1 ounce sour cream

Instructions

For the quesadilla:

1. Prepare a grill for medium-high heat.

2. Sprinkle the chicken with salt and pepper.

3. Grill until cooked through, 12 to 15 minutes, depending on size.

4. Let cool and then shred the chicken into a bowl.

5. Heat the grapeseed oil in a saute pan over medium-high heat.

6. Add the onions and peppers, and cook until caramelized, 8 minutes.

7. Add to the shredded chicken and season with salt and pepper.

8. Lay out the tortillas on a work surface.

9. To one, add the Monterey Jack, followed by the chicken mixture.

10. Top with the Cheddar and cover with the second tortilla.

For the salsa:

1. In a bowl, mix together the onions, tomatoes, lime juice and cilantro.

2. Season with salt and pepper.

3. Heat up the butter in a skillet.

4. Add the pre-made quesadilla and pan-fry until golden.

5. Flip and cook on the reverse side until golden and the cheese is melted.

6. Remove from the pan, cut into 4 wedges and garnish with salsa and sour cream.

Corn and Black Bean Quesadillas

Prepartion time

40 minutes

Ingredients

- Freshly ground black pepper
- Handful of fresh cilantro, chopped
- Eight 8-inch round flour tortillas
- 8 ounces Monterey Jack cheese, shredded
- Pico de gallo, to serve, optional
- 1/4 teaspoon cumin
- 1 to 2 tablespoons olive oil
- 1 medium onion, chopped

- 1 clove garlic, chopped fine
- One 15-ounce can black beans, drained and rinsed
- 1 cup cooked corn kernels (from 1 large ear)
- 3/4 teaspoon salt

Instructions

1. Heat 1 tablespoon of oil in a 10-inch nonstick skillet.

2. Add the onion and garlic; cook until lightly golden, 1 to 2 minutes.

3. Add the beans, corn and another tablespoon of oil if the pan seems dry.

4. Season with the salt, cumin and pepper, and stir in the cilantro.

5. Let cook over medium-low heat until the beans and corn are heated through, about 5 minutes.

6. Heat a 10-inch cast-iron skillet over medium heat.

7. Meanwhile, arrange the tortillas flat on a counter.

8. Sprinkle 1 1/2 tablespoons of cheese on one half of each tortilla.

9. Spoon 2 tablespoons of the bean-corn mixture over the cheese.

10. Top with another 1 1/2 tablespoons of cheese.

11. Fold the filled tortillas into half-moons.

12. Place 2 quesadillas in the skillet.

13. Cook until golden on the bottom and the cheese has started to melt, 2 to 3 minutes.

14. Use a spatula to flip the quesadillas, and cook until golden on the other side, 2 to 3 more minutes,.

15. Repeat with the remaining quesadillas.

16. Serve topped with pico de gallo if desired.

17. Easy Swap In: We usually make the filling with leftover grilled or roasted corn, but frozen corn works great too.

18. Don't thaw the corn-just add the frozen kernels to the pan with the black beans and

allow 1 to 2 extra minutes for them to heat through.

Bulgogi-Inspired Beef Quesadillas

Prepartion time

50 minutes

Ingredients

Pickled Onions:

- 1 red onion, thinly sliced
- 1 cup white vinegar
- 1/4 cup sugar
- 1/4 cup kosher salt

Marinated Beef:

- 1 1/4 cups soy sauce
- 1/2 cup gochujang
- 1/4 cup plus 2 tablespoons sesame oil
- 1/4 cup sesame seeds
- 1/4 cup white vinegar
- 2 tablespoons mirin
- 1 Asian pear, coarsely chopped
- 2 pounds ground beef

To serve:

- 4 tablespoons unsalted butter

- 12 slices American cheese
- Six 10-inch flour tortillas
- 1/2 head iceberg lettuce, shredded
- Sesame seeds, for sprinkling

Instructions

1. For the pickled onions: Combine the onions, vinegar, sugar and salt to in a small saucepan and bring to a boil.

2. Remove from the heat and let cool completely.

3. Drain the pickled onions and set aside.

4. Meanwhile, prepare the beef: Combine the soy sauce, gochujang, sesame oil, sesame

seeds, white vinegar, mirin and Asian pear in a blender and blend until smooth.

5. Pour over the ground beef in a bowl and mix thoroughly.

6. Heat a large, heavy-bottomed skillet over medium-high heat.

7. Add the beef and cook, breaking it up into pieces with a wooden spoon, until browned and cooked through, 8 to 10 minutes.

8. To serve: Heat a large cast-iron skillet over medium heat; add 2 tablespoons of the butter and let melt.

9. Meanwhile, place 2 slices of the American cheese in a tortilla, then top with some of the ground beef, pickled onions and iceberg lettuce.

10. Sprinkle with sesame seeds.

11. Fold the tortilla in half to make a half-moon.

12. Repeat with the remaining ingredients to make 5 more quesadillas.

13. Working in batches, cook the quesadillas in a single layer, adding more butter as needed to the skillet, until golden and crispy on both sides, about 4 minutes per side.

www.ingramcontent.com/pod-product-compliance
Ingram Content Group UK Ltd.
Pitfield, Milton Keynes, MK11 3LW, UK
UKHW022006190726
13853UKWH00004B/1763

9 798529 058374